Mediterranean Diet Cookbook
2021

Family-Friendly, Quick & Easy Recipes to Lose Weight Fast, Live a Healthier Lifestyle, and Regain Confidence

Melinda Barlow

Table of Contents

INTRODUCTION 5
BREKFAST REIPES 8
   1.   Full Eggs in a Squash 8
   2.   Barley Porridge 10
   3.   Tomato and Dill Frittata 11
   4.   Strawberry and Rhubarb Smoothie 13
   5.   Bacon and Brie Omelet Wedges 14
   6.   Pearl Couscous Salad 16
   7.   Coconut Porridge 18
LUNCH RECIPES 20
   8.   Mussels and Veggies Stew 20
   9.   Grapes, Cucumbers and Almonds Soup 22
   10.   Tomato, Sweet Potatoes and Olives Stew 23
   11.   Mint Chicken Soup 24
   12.   Spiced Eggplant Stew 25
   13.   Creamy Salmon Soup 27
   14.   Chicken and Beans Soup 28
DINNER RECIPES 31
   15.   Lamb Chop with Pistachio Gremolata 31
   16.   Pita Salad with Cucumber, Fennel and Chicken 33
   17.   Halibut with Lemon-Fennel Salad 35
   18.   Tuscan Beef Stew 37
   19.   Mediterranean Beef Stew 39
   20.   Cabbage Roll Casserole with Veal 41
   21.   Slow Cooked Daube Provencal 42
MEAT RECIPES 45

22.	Marinated Balsamic Pork Loin Skillet	45
23.	Ground Pork and Beef Chili with Tomato and Basil	47
24.	Warm Beef and Lentil Salad	49
25.	Lighter Lasagna	51
26.	Meatballs in Fresh Tomato Sauce	53
27.	Pork Medallions with Roasted Fennel	55
28.	Stuffed Bell Peppers with Beef and Mushrooms	57

SIDE DISH AND PIZZA RECIPES 60

29.	Basil Bell Peppers and Cucumber Mix	60
30.	Fennel and Walnuts Salad	61
31.	Tomatoes and Black Beans Mix	62
32.	Herbed Beets and Scallions Salad	63
33.	Tomatoes and Endives Mix	64
34.	Yogurt Peppers Mix	65

VEGETARIAN DISHES 67

35.	Summer Vegetables	67
36.	Stir Fried Bok Choy	69
37.	Beans and Cucumber Salad	69
38.	Minty Olives and Tomatoes Salad	71

FISH AND SEAFOOD 73

39.	Ginger Scallion Sauce Over Seared Ahi	73
40.	Healthy Poached Trout	75
41.	Leftover Salmon Salad Power Bowls	76

APPETIZER AND SNACK RECIPES 78

42.	Date Wraps	78
43.	Clementine & Pistachio Ricotta	79
44.	Serrano-Wrapped Plums	80

DESSERT RECIPES 82

| 45. | Italian Bean Soup | 82 |

46.	Red Soup, Seville Style	84
47.	Garlic Soup	86
48.	Dalmatian Cabbage, Potato, And Pea Soup	88
49.	Mini Nuts and Fruits Crumble	90
50.	Mint Banana Chocolate Sorbet	92

INTRODUCTION

A new study has found that intermittent fasting can help you lose weight, and as a result, a vegan diet is more effective at weight loss than a vegetarian or even keto diet. I admit I am a bit confused about the composition of the Mediterranean diet, but it is healthy, easy to keep and it also encourages people to eat more real food in smaller amounts and has a good chance of losing weight - decrease if the changes are permanent. Although this is not a weight loss diet, the study suggests that changing diets from a standard Western diet to a Mediterranean diet could help to lose more weight in the short term.

Many weight loss diets restrict grains, but grains can promote a healthy body weight, and eating whole foods over processed foods is one of the reasons why the Mediterranean diet can help you achieve a healthy weight. Pulses, the most important protein you eat in a Mediterranean diet, can also improve your weight - with the result of losing weight. If you follow a "Mediterranean diet" of dairy, cereals and legumes and do not lose weight, try to minimize your consumption of these things until you notice a reduction or change in these things.

How do I follow a Mediterranean diet plan that is relatively simple, as it does not contain any restrictions to avoid processed foods or sugar and does not require a special cookbook? I have long answered that if you are currently eating a lot of processed food - high in protein, low in carbohydrates - the Mediterranean diet will help you lose body fat, as long as you stick to it consistently and follow it intelligently. Here is a 2,000-calorie daily diet that matches it, similar to the above-mentioned Mediterranean Flexible Diet. I have compiled a list of what is ideal for you to lose weight with your Mediterranean diet, but I will build it from there.

Learn what the Mediterranean diet is, how and why it works, what is Mediterranean in particular and the Cretan cookbook, and have a selection of its meals to help you get started. There is no need to design meals or develop your own steps and weight loss goals, it's all up to you.

Research suggests that the Mediterranean diet could boost weight loss, improve heart health and protect against type 2 diabetes. A review of five studies found that it was more likely to lead to a lower risk of heart disease, diabetes, high blood pressure and high cholesterol. A 2008 study published in the New England Journal of Medicine also showed that weight loss was greater compared to a low-fat diet. Of course, this is not the first time that the Mediterranean diet has been associated with weight loss. In one study, Mediterranean diet groups achieved a 4.5% reduction in body mass index (BMI), which is due to a high protein, low carbohydrate diet and a reduction in cholesterol and blood sugar levels.

This is not the first study to show that the Mediterranean diet is good for people who want to lose weight. In addition to research that highlights its benefits, a recent study has ranked it as one of the best weight loss diets in the world.

The Mediterranean diet is widely recognized as one of the best weight loss diets for people of all ages, races and ethnicities. If you are following the Mediterranean diet to reduce your risk of disease and lose weight, you should fill your eating habits with delicious meals to maintain your motivation on your path to healthier eating.

These eight tips for starting the Mediterranean diet will help you prepare your plate so you can reap the health benefits wherever you start. Click here to learn more about the benefits of the Mediterranean diet for weight loss tips. Try these tips and you will see how you can gain weight and lose weight with your Mediterranean diet. The best tips, tricks and tricks to help you master the European diet, the most popular diet in the world and the best way to master it.

Although these plans often promise rapid weight loss, they can be tempting because they offer dietary rules that can reduce weight - the journey to weight loss feels less overwhelming in the short term. If your primary goal is weight loss and you prefer a Mediterranean diet with a low-fat, high-protein diet, then combining it with weight loss programs like WW can be a great success.

Whether you want to lose weight or just stay healthy, the Mediterranean diet is a well-rounded way to eat without absolute food restrictions. There are simple things you can do to eat the healthy foods that make up a Mediterranean diet.

BREKFAST REIPES

1. Full Eggs in a Squash

Preparation time: 15 minutes

Cooking time: 20 minutes

Servings: 5

Ingredients:

- 2 acorn squash
- 6 whole eggs
- 2 tablespoons extra virgin olive oil
- Salt and pepper as needed
- 5-6 pitted dates
- 8 walnut halves
- A fresh bunch of parsley

Directions:

1. Pre-heat your oven to 375 degrees Fahrenheit. Slice squash crosswise and prepare 3 slices with holes. While slicing the squash, make sure that each slice has a measurement of ¾ inch thickness.
2. Remove the seeds from the slices. Take a baking sheet and line it with parchment paper. Transfer the slices to your baking sheet and season them with salt and pepper.

3. Bake in your oven for 20 minutes. Chop the walnuts and dates on your cutting board. Take the baking dish out of the oven and drizzle slices with olive oil.
4. Crack an egg into each of the holes in the slices and season with pepper and salt. Sprinkle the chopped walnuts on top. Bake for 10 minutes more. Garnish with parsley and add maple syrup.

Nutrition: Calories: 198 Fat: 12g Carbohydrates: 17g Protein: 8g

2. Barley Porridge

Preparation time: 5 minutes

Cooking time: 25 minutes

Servings: 4

Ingredients:

- 1 cup barley
- 1 cup wheat berries
- 2 cups unsweetened almond milk
- 2 cups water
- ½ cup blueberries
- ½ cup pomegranate seeds
- ½ cup hazelnuts, toasted and chopped
- ¼ cup honey

Directions:

1. Take a medium saucepan and place it over medium-high heat. Place barley, almond milk, wheat berries, water and bring to a boil. Reduce the heat to low and simmer for 25 minutes.
2. Divide amongst serving bowls and top each serving with 2 tablespoons blueberries, 2 tablespoons pomegranate seeds, 2 tablespoons hazelnuts, 1 tablespoon honey. Serve and enjoy!

Nutrition: Calories: 295 Fat: 8g Carbohydrates: 56g Protein: 6g

3. Tomato and Dill Frittata

Preparation time: 5 minutes

Cooking time: 10 minutes

Servings: 4

Ingredients:

- 2 tablespoons olive oil
- 1 medium onion, chopped
- 1 teaspoon garlic, minced
- 2 medium tomatoes, chopped
- 6 large eggs
- ½ cup half and half
- ½ cup feta cheese, crumbled
- ¼ cup dill weed
- Salt as needed
- Ground black pepper as needed

Directions:

1. Pre-heat your oven to a temperature of 400 degrees Fahrenheit. Take a large sized ovenproof pan and heat up your olive oil over medium-high heat. Toss in the onion, garlic, tomatoes and stir fry them for 4 minutes.
2. While they are being cooked, take a bowl and beat together your eggs, half and half cream and season the mix with some pepper and salt.
3. Pour the mixture into the pan with your vegetables and top it with crumbled feta cheese and dill weed. Cover it with the lid and let it cook for 3 minutes.

4. Place the pan inside your oven and let it bake for 10 minutes. Serve hot.

Nutrition: Calories: 191 Fat: 15g Carbohydrates: 6g Protein: 9g

4. Strawberry and Rhubarb Smoothie

Preparation time: 5 minutes

Cooking time: 3 minutes

Servings: 1

Ingredients:

- 1 rhubarb stalk, chopped
- 1 cup fresh strawberries, sliced
- ½ cup plain Greek strawberries
- Pinch of ground cinnamon
- 3 ice cubes

Directions:

1. Take a small saucepan and fill with water over high heat. Bring to boil and add rhubarb, boil for 3 minutes. Drain and transfer to blender.
2. Add strawberries, honey, yogurt, cinnamon and pulse mixture until smooth. Add ice cubes and blend until thick with no lumps. Pour into glass and enjoy chilled.

Nutrition: Calories: 295 Fat: 8g Carbohydrates: 56g Protein: 6g

5. Bacon and Brie Omelet Wedges

Preparation time: 10 minutes

Cooking time: 10 minutes

Servings: 6

Ingredients:

- 2 tablespoons olive oil
- 7 ounces smoked bacon
- 6 beaten eggs
- Small bunch chives, snipped
- 3 ½ ounces brie, sliced
- 1 teaspoon red wine vinegar
- 1 teaspoon Dijon mustard
- 1 cucumber, halved, deseeded and sliced diagonally
- 7 ounces radish, quartered

Directions:

1. Turn your grill on and set it to high. Take a small-sized pan and add 1 teaspoon of oil, allow the oil to heat up. Add lardons and fry until crisp. Drain the lardon on kitchen paper.
2. Take another non-sticky cast iron frying pan and place it over grill, heat 2 teaspoons of oil. Add lardons, eggs, chives, ground pepper to the frying pan. Cook on low until they are semi-set.
3. Carefully lay brie on top and grill until the Brie sets and is a golden texture. Remove it from the pan and cut up into wedges.

4. Take a small bowl and create dressing by mixing olive oil, mustard, vinegar and seasoning. Add cucumber to the bowl and mix, serve alongside the omelet wedges.

Nutrition: Calories: 35 Fat: 31g Carbohydrates: 3g Protein: 25g

6. Pearl Couscous Salad

Preparation time: 15 minutes

Cooking time: 0 minutes

Servings: 6

Ingredients:

- For Lemon Dill Vinaigrette:
- Juice of 1 large sized lemon
- 1/3 cup of extra virgin olive oil
- 1 teaspoon of dill weed
- 1 teaspoon of garlic powder
- Salt as needed
- Pepper
- For Israeli Couscous:
- 2 cups of Pearl Couscous
- Extra virgin olive oil
- 2 cups of halved grape tomatoes
- Water as needed
- 1/3 cup of finely chopped red onions
- ½ of a finely chopped English cucumber
- 15 ounces of chickpeas
- 14 ounce can of artichoke hearts (roughly chopped up)
- ½ cup of pitted Kalamata olives
- 15-20 pieces of fresh basil leaves, roughly torn and chopped up
- 3 ounces of fresh baby mozzarella

Directions:

1. Prepare the vinaigrette by taking a bowl and add the ingredients listed under vinaigrette. Mix them well and keep aside. Take a medium-sized heavy pot and place it over medium heat.
2. Add 2 tablespoons of olive oil and allow it to heat up. Add couscous and keep cooking until golden brown. Add 3 cups of boiling water and cook the couscous according to the package instructions.
3. Once done, drain in a colander and keep aside. Take another large-sized mixing bowl and add the remaining ingredients except the cheese and basil.
4. Add the cooked couscous and basil to the mix and mix everything well. Give the vinaigrette a nice stir and whisk it into the couscous salad. Mix well.
5. Adjust the seasoning as required. Add mozzarella cheese. Garnish with some basil. Enjoy!

Nutrition: Calories: 393 Fat: 13g Carbohydrates: 57g Protein: 13g

7. Coconut Porridge

Preparation time: 15 minutes

Cooking time: 0 minutes

Servings: 6

Ingredients:

- Powdered erythritol as needed
- 1 ½ cups almond milk, unsweetened
- 2 tablespoons vanilla protein powder
- 3 tablespoons Golden Flaxseed meal
- 2 tablespoons coconut flour

Directions:

1. Take a bowl and mix in flaxseed meal, protein powder, coconut flour and mix well. Add mix to saucepan (placed over medium heat).
2. Add almond milk and stir, let the mixture thicken. Add your desired amount of sweetener and serve. Enjoy!

Nutrition: Calories: 259 Fat: 13g Carbohydrates: 5g Protein: 16g

LUNCH RECIPES

8. Mussels and Veggies Stew

Preparation time: 10 minutes

Cooking time: 30 minutes

Servings: 4

Ingredients:

- 1 yellow onion, chopped
- 2 tablespoons olive oil
- 1 fennel bulb, chopped
- 1 carrot, chopped
- 1 red bell pepper, chopped
- 2 garlic cloves, minced
- 3 tablespoons tomato paste
- 16 ounces canned chickpeas, drained
- 1 teaspoon thyme, dried
- ¼ teaspoon smoked paprika
- Salt and black pepper to the taste
- 3 and ½ cups water
- 1-pound mussels, scrubbed

Directions:

1. Heat up a pot with the oil over medium high heat, add the fennel, onion, bell pepper and carrot, stir and cook for 5 minutes.

2. Add the garlic and tomato paste, stir and cook for 1 minute more.
3. Add the rest of the ingredients except the mussels, stir, bring to a simmer and cook for 20 minutes.
4. Add the mussels, cook the stew for 4-5 minutes more, divide into bowls and serve.

Nutrition: calories 450, fat 12, fiber 13, carbs 47, protein 34

9. Grapes, Cucumbers and Almonds Soup

Preparation time: 10 minutes

Cooking time: 0 minutes

Servings: 4

Ingredients:

- ¼ cup almonds, chopped and toasted
- 3 cucumbers, peeled and chopped
- 3 garlic cloves, minced
- ½ cup warm water
- 6 scallions, sliced
- ¼ cup white wine vinegar
- 3 tablespoons olive oil
- Salt and white pepper to the taste
- 1 teaspoon lemon juice
- ½ cup green grapes, halved

Directions:

1. In your blender, combine the almonds with the cucumbers and the rest of the ingredients except the grapes and lemon juice, pulse well and divide into bowls.
2. Top each serving with the lemon juice and grapes and serve cold.

Nutrition: calories 200, fat 5.4, fiber 2.4, carbs 7.6, protein 3.3

10. Tomato, Sweet Potatoes and Olives Stew

Preparation time: 10 minutes

Cooking time: 30 minutes

Servings: 4

Ingredients:

- 1 yellow onion, chopped
- 1 tablespoon olive oil
- 2 cups sweet potatoes, peeled and chopped
- 1 and ½ teaspoon cumin, ground
- 20 ounces canned tomatoes, chopped
- 1 and ½ teaspoon honey
- 6 tablespoons orange juice
- 1 cup water
- Salt and black pepper to the taste
- ½ cup green olives, pitted and halved
- 1 tablespoon cilantro, chopped

Directions:

1. Heat up a pot with the oil over medium heat, add the onion, stir and sauté for 5 minutes.
2. Add the rest of the ingredients, stir, bring to a simmer and cook over medium heat for 25 minutes.
3. Divide the stew into bowls and serve.

Nutrition: calories 235, fat 12.3, fiber 3.5, carbs 16.3, protein 10.2

11. Mint Chicken Soup

Preparation time: 10 minutes

Cooking time: 30 minutes

Servings: 4

Ingredients:

- Salt and black pepper to the taste
- 6 cups chicken stock
- ¼ cup lemon juice
- 1 chicken breast, boneless, skinless and cubed
- ½ cup white rice
- 6 tablespoons mint, chopped

Directions:

1. Put the stock in a pot, add salt and pepper, bring to a simmer over medium heat, add the rice and cook for 15 minutes.
2. Add the rest of the ingredients, stir, cook for 15 minutes more, divide into bowls and serve.

Nutrition: calories 232, fat 11, fiber 2.4, carbs 14.3, protein 12.4

12. Spiced Eggplant Stew

Preparation time: 10 minutes

Cooking time: 45 minutes

Servings: 4

Ingredients:

- 4 eggplants, cubed
- Salt and black pepper to the taste
- 2 yellow onions, chopped
- 2 red bell peppers, chopped
- 30 ounces canned tomatoes, chopped
- 1 cup black olives, pitted and chopped
- ¼ teaspoon allspice, ground
- ½ teaspoon cinnamon powder
- 1 teaspoon oregano, dried
- A drizzle of olive oil
- A pinch of red chili flakes
- 3 tablespoons Greek yogurt

Directions:

1. Heat up a pot with the oil over medium high heat, add the onions, bell pepper, oregano, cinnamon and the allspice and sauté for 5 minutes.
2. Add the rest of the ingredients except the flakes and the yogurt, bring to a simmer and cook over medium heat for 40 minutes.
3. Divide the stew into bowls, top each serving with the flakes and the yogurt and serve.

Nutrition: calories 256, fat 3.5, fiber 25.4, carbs 53.3, protein 8.8

13. Creamy Salmon Soup

Preparation time: 10 minutes

Cooking time: 15 minutes

Servings: 6

Ingredients:

- 2 tablespoon olive oil
- 1 red onion, chopped
- Salt and white pepper to the taste
- 3 gold potatoes, peeled and cubed
- 2 carrots, chopped
- 4 cups fish stock
- 4 ounces salmon fillets, boneless and cubed
- ½ cup heavy cream
- 1 tablespoon dill, chopped

Directions:

1. Heat up a pan with the oil over medium heat, add the onion, and sauté for 5 minutes.
2. Add the rest of the ingredients expect the cream, salmon and the dill, bring to a simmer and cook for 5-6 minutes more.
3. Add the salmon, cream and the dill, simmer for 5 minutes more, divide into bowls and serve.

Nutrition: calories 214, fat 16.3, fiber 1.5, carbs 6.4, protein 11.8

14. Chicken and Beans Soup

Preparation time: 10 minutes

Cooking time: 1 hour

Servings: 6

Ingredients:

- 2 tablespoons olive oil
- 2 yellow onions, chopped
- 3 tomatoes, chopped
- 4 cups chicken stock
- 1-pound chicken breasts, skinless, boneless and cubed
- 3 garlic cloves, minced
- 3 red chili peppers, chopped
- 1 tablespoon coriander seeds, crushed
- 14 ounces canned black beans, drained
- Zest of 1 lime, grated
- Juice of 1 lime
- Salt and black pepper to the taste
- 1 tablespoon coriander, chopped

Directions:

1. Heat up a pot with the oil over medium heat, add the onions, the chicken, garlic, chili peppers and the coriander and sauté for 10 minutes.
2. Add the rest of the ingredients, bring to a simmer over medium heat, cook for 50 minutes, ladle into bowls and serve.

Nutrition: calories 667, fat 17.6, fiber 17.6, carbs 72.3, protein 55.4

DINNER RECIPES

15. Lamb Chop with Pistachio Gremolata

Preparation Time: 10 minutes

Cooking Time: 8 minutes

Serving: 4

Ingredients:

- 8 trimmed lamb loin chops
- 2 tbsp chopped flat-leaf parsley
- 2 tbsp finely chopped pistachios
- 1 tbsp chopped cilantro
- 2 tsp grated lemon zest
- ½ tsp salt
- ½ tsp ground cumin
- ¼ tsp ground coriander
- ¼ tsp black pepper
- 1/8 tsp salt
- 1/8 ground cinnamon
- 1 clove minced garlic

Direction:

1. Heat nonstick pan at medium-high heat. Combine the cumin, coriander, cinnamon, salt and black pepper and season evenly on both sides of the lamb. Grease the pan with cooking spray and add the lamb, cook for 4 min per side.

2. In the meantime, combine the pistachios, cilantro, parsley, lemon zest, salt and garlic, season over the lamb.

Nutrition: 409 Calories 41g Protein 22g Fat

16. Pita Salad with Cucumber, Fennel and Chicken

Preparation Time: 10 minutes

Cooking Time: 12 minutes

Serving: 4

Ingredients:

- 2 (6-inch) pitas
- ½ halved lengthwise and thinly sliced English cucumber
- 2 cups thinly sliced fennel bulb
- 1 cup shredded skinless, boneless rotisserie chicken breast
- ½ cup chopped flat-leaf parsley
- ¼ cup vertically sliced red onion
- ¼ cup lemon juice
- 3 tbsp extra-virgin olive oil
- 1 tbsp white wine vinegar
- ½ tsp chopped oregano
- ½ tsp salt, divided
- ¼ tsp black pepper, divided

Direction:

1. Preheat the oven to 350°F.
2. Situate pitas on a baking tray and bake for 12 min, cool down 1 min. Cut into small pieces and combine with fennel, chicken, parsley and red onion. Season with ¼ tsp of salt and 1/8 tsp of pepper.

3. Add the juice, oregano, vinegar, the remaining ¼ tsp of salt and 1/8 tsp of pepper. Gradually add the oil, mixing with a whisk. Season with dressing over the pita mixture to coat and serve.

Nutrition: 413 Calories 38g Protein 17g Fat

17. Halibut with Lemon-Fennel Salad

Preparation Time: 15 minutes

Cooking Time: 5 minutes

Serving: 4

Ingredients:

- 4 halibut fillets
- 2 cups thinly sliced fennel bulb
- ¼ cup thinly vertically sliced red onion
- 2 tbsp lemon juice
- 1 tbsp thyme leaves
- 1 tbsp chopped flat-leaf parsley
- 5 tsp extra-virgin olive oil, divided
- 1 tsp coriander
- ½ tsp salt
- ½ tsp cumin
- ¼ tsp ground black pepper
- 2 cloves minced garlic

Direction:

1. Combine the coriander, cumin, salt and black pepper in a small bowl. Combine 2 tsp of olive oil, garlic and 1 ½ tsp of spice mixture in another small bowl, evenly rub the garlic mixture on the halibut. Heat 1 tsp of oil in a large nonstick pan over medium-high heat. Cook the halibut to the pan for 5 min.
2. Combine the remaining 2 tsp of oil, ¾ tsp of spice mixture, the fennel bulb, onion, lemon juice, thyme

leaves and parsley in a bowl, mix well to coat, and serve salad with halibut.

Nutrition: 427 Calories 39g Protein 20g Fat

18. Tuscan Beef Stew

Preparation Time 10 minutes

Cooking Time 4 hours

Serving: 8

Ingredients

- 2 pounds beef stew meat
- 4 carrots
- 2 (14½-ounce) cans tomatoes
- 1 medium onion
- 1 package McCormick Slow Cookers Hearty Beef Stew Seasoning
- ½ cup water
- ½ cup dry red wine
- 1 teaspoon rosemary leaves
- 8 slices Italian bread

Directions

1. Place the cubed beef in the slow cooker along with the carrots, diced tomatoes, and onion wedges.
2. Mix the seasoning package in the ½ cup of water and stir well, making sure there are no lumps remaining.
3. Add the red wine to the water and stir slightly. Add the rosemary leaves to the water-and-wine mixture and then pour over the meat, stirring to ensure the meat is completely covered.
4. Switch the slow cooker to low then cook for 8 hours, or cook for 4 hours on high.

5. Serve with toasted Italian bread.

Nutrition: 329 Calories 15g fat 25.6g protein

19. Mediterranean Beef Stew

Preparation Time 25 minutes

Cooking Time 8 hours

Serving: 6

Ingredients

- 1 tablespoon olive oil
- 8 ounces sliced mushrooms
- 1 onion
- 2 pounds chuck roast
- 1 cup beef stock
- 1 (14½-ounce) can tomatoes with juice
- ½ cup tomato sauce
- ¼ cup balsamic vinegar
- 1 can black olives
- ½ cup garlic cloves
- 2 tablespoons fresh rosemary
- 2 tablespoons fresh parsley
- 1 tablespoon capers

Directions

- Heat a skillet over high heat. Add 1 tablespoon of olive oil. Once heated, cook cubed roast.
- Once cooked, stir rest of the olive oil (if needed), then toss in the onions and mushrooms. When they have softened, transfer to the slow cooker.
- Add the beef stock to the skillet to deglaze the pan, then pour it over the meat in the slow cooker.

- Mix rest of the ingredients to the slow cooker to coat.
- Set the temperature on your slow cooker to low and cook for 8 hours.

Nutrition: 471 Calories 23.4g fat 47.1g protein

20. Cabbage Roll Casserole with Veal

Preparation Time 5 minutes

Cooking Time 4–8 hours

Serving: 6

Ingredients

- 1-pound raw ground veal
- 1 head of cabbage
- 1 medium green pepper
- 1 medium onion, chopped
- 1 (15-ounce) can tomatoes
- 2 (15-ounce) cans tomato sauce
- 1 teaspoon minced garlic
- 1 tablespoon Worcestershire sauce
- 1 tablespoon beef bouillon
- ½ teaspoon salt
- ½ teaspoon pepper
- 1 cup uncooked brown rice

Directions

1. Situate all the ingredients to your slow cooker
2. Stir well to combine.
3. Adjust your slow cooker to high and cook for 4 hours, or cook for 8 hours on low.

Nutrition: 335 Calories 18g fat 22.9g protein

21. Slow Cooked Daube Provencal

Preparation Time 15 minutes

Cooking Time: 4–8 hours

Serving: 8–10

Ingredients

- 1 tablespoon olive oil
- 10 garlic cloves, minced
- 2 pounds boneless chuck roast
- 1½ teaspoons salt
- ½ teaspoon black pepper
- 1 cup dry red wine
- 2 cups carrots, chopped
- 1½ cups onion, chopped
- ½ cup beef broth
- 1 (14-ounce) can diced tomatoes
- 1 tablespoon tomato paste
- 1 teaspoon fresh rosemary, chopped
- 1 teaspoon fresh thyme, chopped
- ½ teaspoon orange zest, grated
- ½ teaspoon ground cinnamon
- ¼ teaspoon ground cloves
- 1 bay leaf

Directions

1. Preheat skillet and then add the olive oil. Cook minced garlic and onions

2. Add the cubed meat, salt, and pepper and cook until the meat has browned.
3. Transfer the meat to the slow cooker.
4. Put beef broth to the skillet and let simmer for about 3 minutes to deglaze the pan, then pour into slow cooker over the meat.
5. Incorporate the rest of the ingredients to the slow cooker and stir well to combine.
6. Adjust your slow cooker to low and cook for 8 hours, or set to high and cook for 4 hours.
7. Serve with a side of egg noodles, rice or some crusty Italian bread.

Nutrition: 547 Calories 30.5g fat 45.2g protein

MEAT RECIPES

22. Marinated Balsamic Pork Loin Skillet

Preparation Time: 20 minutes

Cooking Time: 15 minutes

Servings: 4-6

Ingredients:

- 1 lb. pork tenderloin, sliced ½" thick
- 1/4 cup balsamic vinegar
- 1/4 cup extra virgin olive oil
- 1/2 teaspoon smoked paprika or regular paprika
- 1 tablespoon honey (optional)
- 1/2 teaspoon minced garlic
- Salt and pepper, to taste
- 1/4 teaspoon oregano
- 1/4 teaspoon dried marjoram or rosemary
- 1 cup sliced red onion
- 2 oz. sliced olives
- 1 zucchini, thinly sliced
- Fresh basil
- To serve…
- Paprika or red pepper flakes
- Mixed leafy greens

Directions:

1. Grab a large bowl and add the balsamic marinade ingredients then stir well to combine.
2. Place the lamb into the bowl, stir well then pop into the fridge for at least 30 minutes to marinate.
3. When you're ready to start cooking, place a skillet over a medium heat. Add a drop of oil to prevent sticking then add the onion and cook for 5 minutes until soft.
4. Add the pork loin and remaining marinade, stir well then cook on medium for 5 minutes.
5. Flip the pork and add the olive and zucchini.
6. Cook for 5 minutes more until the pork is no longer pink.
7. Serve and enjoy.

Nutrition: Calories: 309 Net carbs: 7g Fat: 19g Protein: 26g

23. Ground Pork and Beef Chili with Tomato and Basil

Preparation Time: 10 minutes

Cooking Time: 20 minutes

Servings: 5

Ingredients:

- 3 Tbsp. olive oil
- 1 large onion, finely chopped
- 5 garlic cloves, finely chopped
- 1 tsp. dried red chili flakes
- 2 red bell peppers, finely chopped
- 1 lb. ground beef
- 1 lb. ground pork
- ½ cup red wine
- 3 cups canned chopped tomatoes
- ½ cup roughly chopped fresh basil
- Salt and pepper

Directions:

1. Add the olive oil to a large sauté pan over a medium-high heat
2. Add the onions, garlic, chili, and bell peppers and stir as they soften together, for about 3 minutes
3. Add the pork and beef and stir as they turn from pink to brown
4. Add the wine and allow the alcohol to burn off for about 2 minutes

5. Add the tomatoes, basil, salt and pepper, cover and allow to simmer for about 15 minutes. If it appears to be drying out, add a little water!
6. Serve hot, with brown rice pasta, or a side salad

Nutrition: Calories: 589 Fat: 36.9 grams Protein: 44.5 grams Total carbs: 14.4 grams Net carbs: 12.5 grams

24. Warm Beef and Lentil Salad

Preparation Time: 10 minutes

Cooking Time: 15 minutes

Servings: 4

Ingredients:

- 1 large piece of steak, (rump steak is great), about 1 lb., room temperature
- 1 Tbsp. olive oil
- Salt and pepper
- 3 cups canned brown lentils, (3 cups once drained)
- ½ red onion, finely chopped
- 3 oz. feta cheese, crumbled
- ½ cup finely chopped parsley
- 1/3 cup finely chopped mint
- Juice of 1 lemon
- 3 Tbsp. olive oil

Directions:

1. Place a skillet over a high heat
2. Rub the steak with olive oil and sprinkle with salt and pepper
3. Lay the steak onto the hot skillet and sear on both sides until golden, but still blushing in the center (medium rare), leave to rest while you prepare the salad
4. In a large salad bowl, toss the lentils, onion, feta, parsley, mint, lemon juice, and olive oil

5. Slice the warm steak into thin slices and lay on top of the salad, or divide individually when serving

Nutrition: Calories: 442 Fat: 21.3 grams Protein: 39.3 grams Total carbs: 24.8 grams Net carbs: 18.4 grams

25. Lighter Lasagna

Preparation Time: 20 minutes

Cooking Time: 1 hour

Servings: 6

Ingredients:

- 2 Tbsp. olive oil
- 1 onion, finely chopped
- 4 garlic cloves, finely chopped
- 1 ½ lbs. ground beef
- 1/3 Cup red wine
- 2 cups canned chopped tomatoes
- 1 tsp. dried chili flakes
- 1 tsp. each dried oregano, thyme, and rosemary
- Salt and pepper
- 12 sheets (12 halves or 6 whole sheets) fresh lasagna (enough to create three layers across the entire dish)
- Large handful of fresh basil
- 5 oz. fresh Mozzarella, torn

Directions:

1. Add the olive oil to a large sauté pan over a medium-high heat
2. Add the onion and garlic to the pan and stir as they soften for about 2 minutes
3. Add the beef and stir as it turns from pink to brown
4. Add the red wine and allow the alcohol to burn off for about 2 minutes

5. Add the tomatoes, chili flakes, herbs, salt and pepper and stir to combine
6. Leave to simmer for about 30 minutes until thick and rich in flavor
7. Preheat the oven to 400 degrees Fahrenheit and have a lasagna dish waiting by
8. Layer the lasagna in this fashion: start with a layer of beef mixture on the bottom, then a layer of pasta, then a few torn basil leaves, repeat until everything has been used, and the top layer is beef sauce (it's not meant to be super tidy, just throw it all together as you please, as long as it's roughly even!)
9. Finish with the torn Mozzarella and a few extra basil leaves
10. Bake in the oven for about 30 minutes or until everything is golden and bubbling

Nutrition: Calories: 714 Fat: 34 grams Protein: 50.5 grams Total carbs: 47.1 grams Net carbs: 41 grams

26. Meatballs in Fresh Tomato Sauce

Preparation Time: 15 minutes

Cooking Time: 25 minutes

Servings: 4

Ingredients:

- Meatballs:
- 4 garlic cloves, crushed
- 1 onion, finely chopped
- 1 lb. ground beef
- 1 tsp. each dried oregano, thyme, and rosemary
- 1 egg
- ½ cup whole grain bread crumbs
- Salt and pepper
- Sauce:
- 2 Tbsp. olive oil
- 2 garlic cloves
- ½ onion, finely chopped
- ½ cup red wine
- 8 fresh tomatoes, chopped
- 2 Tbsp. pure tomato paste
- ½ fresh red chili, finely chopped (optional)
- Salt and pepper
- ½ cup beef stock or water
- To serve:
- ½ cup dried whole grain pasta (per serving), boiled in salty water until soft, but with a little "bite"
- 1 cup broccoli (per serving), steamed

Directions:
1. Preheat the oven to 380 degrees F and line a baking tray with baking paper
2. In a large bowl combine all of the meatball ingredients with clean hands, or a very sturdy wooden spoon
3. Roll the meatball mixture into golf ball-sized balls and place them onto the lined tray, pop the tray into the oven and cook the meatballs for about 25 minutes, turning once, until golden all around
4. Drizzle the olive oil into a large sauté pan over a medium-high heat
5. Add the garlic and onions to the pan and allow them to soften, as you stir, for about 2 minutes
6. Add the wine to the pan and allow to reduce for a few minutes
7. Add the tomatoes, tomato paste, chili, salt, and pepper and stir to combine
8. Allow the sauce to simmer and become rich for about 5 minutes, adding a little water or beef stock if it appears to be drying out
9. Add the cooked meatballs to the sauté pan and drench them in sauce
10. Serve the meatballs on sauce on a small bed of whole grain pasta, with steamed broccoli on the side

Nutrition: Calories: 610 Fat: 22.4 grams Protein: 38.1 grams Total carbs: 64.9 grams Net carbs: 54.2 grams

27. Pork Medallions with Roasted Fennel

Preparation Time: 15 minutes

Cooking Time: 30 minutes

Servings: 4

Ingredients:

- 4 pork medallions
- 2 Tbsp. olive oil
- 1 sprig fresh thyme
- 1 sprig fresh rosemary
- Salt and pepper
- 1 lb. fennel bulbs, cut into quarters, (lengthwise)
- 3 Tbsp. olive oil
- Salt and pepper

Directions:

1. Preheat the oven to 450 degrees F and line a baking tray with baking paper
2. Lay the fennel bulb. quarters onto the tray and rub with olive oil, salt and pepper. Slip the tray into the oven and roast the fennel for 30 minutes, turning once. We're aiming for soft, slightly caramelized, golden fennel quarters!
3. As the fennel is roasting: place a large skillet over a high medium-heat
4. Lay the pork medallions onto a large board and use a wooden spoon to gently "bash" them

5. Rub the pork on both sides with olive oil and sprinkle with salt and pepper
6. Lay the pork medallions onto the hot pan, nestle the thyme and rosemary between them, and sear on both sides for about 2 minutes or until each side is golden and the meat is cooked through but still juicy
7. Let the pork rest for a few minutes before serving with roasted fennel!

Nutrition: Calories: 439 Fat: 20.2 grams Protein: 37.2 grams Total carbs: 8.3 grams Net carbs: 4.8 grams

28. Stuffed Bell Peppers with Beef and Mushrooms

Preparation Time: 10 minutes

Cooking Time: 20 minutes

Servings: 4

Ingredients:

- 4 large red bell peppers, halved, seeds removed
- 1 Tbsp. olive oil
- 2 garlic cloves, finely chopped
- 1 onion, finely chopped
- 1 lb. ground beef
- 4 large Portobello mushrooms, finely chopped
- 1 tomato, finely chopped
- 1 tsp. each dried thyme, oregano, and rosemary
- Salt and pepper
- Parmesan cheese (about 2 oz.)

Directions:

1. Preheat the oven to 400 degrees Fahrenheit and line a baking tray with baking paper
2. Prep the bell peppers and lay them on the lined tray, set aside
3. Drizzle the olive oil into a large sauté pan over a medium-high heat
4. Add the garlic and onion and stir as they soften for a minute or two

5. Add the beef and mushrooms, stir to combine, and allow the beef to turn from pink to brown
6. Add the tomatoes, herbs, salt and pepper to the meat, stir, and leave to simmer for about 10 minutes. (Note: the beef and mushroom mixture will likely be quite wet, which is fine!)
7. Spoon the beef mixture into the awaiting bell pepper halves and grate a small scattering of parmesan cheese over each one
8. Bake for about 20 minutes or until the peppers are soft!

Nutrition: Calories: 363 Fat: 16.3 grams Protein: 33.7 grams Total carbs: 19.6 grams Net carbs: 13.2 grams

SIDE DISH AND PIZZA RECIPES

29. Basil Bell Peppers and Cucumber Mix

Preparation time: 5 minutes

Cooking time: 0 minutes

Servings: 6

Ingredients:

- 1 red bell pepper, cut into strips
- 1 green bell pepper, cut into strips
- 2 cucumbers, sliced
- ½ cup balsamic vinegar
- 2 tablespoons olive oil
- 1 tablespoon sesame seeds, toasted
- 1 tablespoon basil, chopped

Directions:

1. In a bowl, combine the bell peppers with the cucumber and the rest of the ingredients except the sesame seeds and toss.
2. Sprinkle the sesame seeds, divide the mix between plates and serve as a side dish.

Nutrition: calories 226, fat 8.7, fiber 3.4, carbs 14.4, protein 5.6

30. Fennel and Walnuts Salad

Preparation time: 5 minutes

Cooking time: 0 minutes

Servings: 4

Ingredients:

- 8 dates, pitted and sliced
- 2 fennel bulbs, sliced
- 2 tablespoons chives, chopped
- ½ cup walnuts, chopped
- 2 tablespoons lime juice
- 2 tablespoons olive oil
- Salt and black pepper to the taste

Directions:

1. In a salad bowl, combine the fennel with dates and the rest of the ingredients, toss, divide between plates and serve as a side salad.

Nutrition: calories 200, fat 7.6, fiber 2.4, carbs 14.5, protein 4.3

31. Tomatoes and Black Beans Mix

Preparation time: 10 minutes

Cooking time: 0 minutes

Servings: 4

Ingredients:

- 15 ounces canned black beans, drained and rinsed
- 1 cup cherry tomatoes, halved
- 2 spring onions, chopped
- 3 tablespoons olive oil
- 1 and ½ teaspoons orange zest, grated
- 1 teaspoon honey
- Salt and black pepper to the taste
- ½ teaspoon cumin, ground
- 1 tablespoon lime juice

Directions:

1. In a bowl, combine the beans with cherry tomatoes, onions and the rest of the ingredients, toss and keep in the fridge for 10 minutes before serving as a side dish.

Nutrition: calories 284, fat 7.5, fiber 15.3, carbs 25.5, protein 12.4

32. Herbed Beets and Scallions Salad

Preparation time: 10 minutes

Cooking time: 0 minutes

Servings: 8

Ingredients:

- 4 red beets, cooked, peeled and sliced
- 6 scallions, chopped
- Zest of 1 lemon, grated
- 2 cups mixed basil with mint, parsley and cilantro, chopped
- ¼ cup balsamic vinegar
- 2 teaspoons poppy seeds
- 1 and ½ tablespoons olive oil
- Salt and black pepper to the taste

Directions:

1. In a salad bowl, combine the beets with the scallions, lemon zest and the rest of the ingredients, toss, keep in the fridge for 10 minutes and serve as a side salad.

Nutrition: calories 283, fat 11.4, fiber 3.5, carbs 13.5, protein 6.5

33. Tomatoes and Endives Mix

Preparation time: 10 minutes

Cooking time: 20 minutes

Servings: 4

Ingredients:

- 4 endives, shredded
- 14 ounces canned tomatoes, chopped
- Salt and black pepper to the taste
- 2 garlic cloves, minced
- ½ teaspoon red pepper, crushed
- 3 tablespoons olive oil
- 1 tablespoon oregano, chopped
- 2 tablespoons parmesan, grated
- 1 tablespoon cilantro, chopped

Directions:

1. Heat up a pan with the oil over medium heat, add the garlic and the red pepper and cook for 2-3 minutes.
2. Add the endives, tomatoes, salt, pepper and the oregano, stir and sauté for 15 minutes more.
3. Add the remaining ingredients, toss, cook for 2 minutes, divide the mix between plates and serve as a side dish.

Nutrition: calories 232, fat 7.5, fiber 3.5, carbs 14.3, protein 4.5

34. Yogurt Peppers Mix

Preparation time: 10 minutes

Cooking time: 15 minutes

Servings: 4

Ingredients:

- 2 red bell peppers, cut into thick strips
- 2 tablespoons olive oil
- 3 shallots, chopped
- 3 garlic cloves, minced
- Salt and black pepper to the taste
- ½ cup Greek yogurt
- 1 tablespoon cilantro, chopped

Directions:

1. Heat up a pan with the oil over medium heat, add the shallots and garlic, stir and cook for 5 minutes.
2. Add the rest of the ingredients, toss, cook for 10 minutes more, divide the mix between plates and serve as a side dish.

Nutrition: calories 274, fat 11, fiber 3.5, protein 13.3, carbs 6.5

VEGETARIAN DISHES

35. Summer Vegetables

Preparation Time: 20 minutes

Cooking Time: 1 hour 40 minutes minute

Servings: 6

Ingredients:

- 1 tsp. dried marjoram
- 1/3 cup Parmesan cheese
- 1 small eggplant, sliced into ¼-inch thick circles
- 1 small summer squash, peeled and sliced diagonally into ¼-inch thickness
- 3 large tomatoes, sliced into ¼-inch thick circles
- ½ cup dry white wine
- ½ tsp. freshly ground pepper, divided
- ½ tsp. salt, divided
- 5 cloves garlic, sliced thinly
- 2 cups leeks, sliced thinly
- 4 tbsp. extra virgin olive oil, divided

Directions:

1. On medium fire, place a large nonstick saucepan and heat 2 tbsp. oil.
2. Sauté garlic and leeks for 6 minutes or until garlic is starting to brown. Season with pepper and salt, ¼ tsp. each.

3. Pour in wine and cook for another minute. Transfer to a 2-quart baking dish.
4. In baking dish, layer in alternating pattern the eggplant, summer squash, and tomatoes. Do this until dish is covered with vegetables. If there are excess vegetables, store for future use.
5. Season with remaining pepper and salt. Drizzle with remaining olive oil and pop in a preheated 425oF oven.
6. Bake for 75 minutes. Remove from oven and top with marjoram and cheese.
7. Return to oven and bake for 15 minutes more or until veggies are soft and edges are browned.
8. Allow to cool for at least 5 minutes before serving.

Nutrition: Calories: 150; Carbs: 11.8g; Protein: 3.3g; Fat: 10.8g

36. Stir Fried Bok Choy

Preparation Time: 5 minutes

Cooking Time: 13 minutes

Servings: 4

Ingredients:

- 3 tbsp. coconut oil
- 4 cloves of garlic, minced
- 1 onion, chopped
- 2 heads bok choy, rinsed and chopped
- 2 tsp. coconut aminos
- Salt and pepper to taste
- 2 tbsp. sesame oil
- 2 tbsp. sesame seeds, toasted

Directions:

1. Heat the oil in a pot for 2 minutes.
2. Sauté the garlic and onions until fragrant, around 3 minutes.
3. Stir in the bok choy, coconut aminos, salt and pepper.
4. Cover pan and cook for 5 minutes.
5. Stir and continue cooking for another 3 minutes.
6. Drizzle with sesame oil and sesame seeds on top before serving.

Nutrition: Calories: 358; Carbs: 5.2g; Protein: 21.5g; Fat: 28.4g

37. Beans and Cucumber Salad

Preparation Time: 10 minutes

Cooking Time: 0 minutes

Servings: 4

Ingredients:

- 15 oz. canned great northern beans, drained and rinsed
- 2 tbsp. olive oil
- ½ cup baby arugula
- 1 cup cucumber, sliced
- 1 tbsp. parsley, chopped
- 2 tomatoes, cubed
- A pinch of sea salt and black pepper
- 2 tbsp. balsamic vinegar

Directions:

1. In a bowl, mix the beans with the cucumber and the rest of the ingredients, toss and serve cold.

Nutrition: Calories 233, Fat 9g, Fiber 6.5g, Carbs 13g, Protein 8g

38. Minty Olives and Tomatoes Salad

Preparation Time: 10 minutes

Cooking Time: 0 minutes

Servings: 4

Ingredients:

- 1 cup kalamata olives, pitted and sliced
- 1 cup black olives, pitted and halved
- 1 cup cherry tomatoes, halved
- 4 tomatoes, chopped
- 1 red onion, chopped
- 2 tbsp. oregano, chopped
- 1 tbsp. mint, chopped
- 2 tbsp. balsamic vinegar
- ¼ cup olive oil
- 2 tsp. Italian herbs, dried
- A pinch of sea salt and black pepper

Directions:

1. In a salad bowl, mix the olives with the tomatoes and the rest of the ingredients, toss and serve cold.

Nutrition: Calories 190, Fat 8.1g, Fiber 5.8g, Carbs 11.6g, Protein 4.6g

FISH AND SEAFOOD

39. Ginger Scallion Sauce Over Seared Ahi

Preparation Time: 10 Minutes

Cooking Time: 6 Minutes

Servings: 4

Ingredients:

- 1 Bunch Scallions, Bottoms Removed, Finely Chopped
- 1 Tbsp. Rice Wine Vinegar
- 1 Tbsp. Bragg's Liquid Amino
- 16-Oz Ahi Tuna Steaks
- 2 Tbsp. Fresh Ginger, Peeled And Grated
- 3 Tbsp. Coconut Oil, Melted
- Pepper And Salt To Taste

Directions:

1. In A Small Bowl Mix Together Vinegar, 2 Tbsp. Oil, Soy Sauce, Ginger And Scallions. Put Aside.
2. On Medium Fire, Place A Large Saucepan And Heat Remaining Oil. Once Oil Is Hot And Starts To Smoke, Sear Tuna Until Deeply Browned Or For Two Minutes Per Side.
3. Place Seared Tuna On A Serving Platter And Let It Stand For 5 Minutes Before Slicing Into 1-Inch-Thick Strips.

4. Drizzle Ginger-Scallion Mixture Over Seared Tuna, Serve And Enjoy.

Nutrition: Calories: 247; Protein: 29g; Fat: 1g; Carbs: 8g

40. Healthy Poached Trout

Preparation Time: 10 minutes

Cooking Time: 10 minutes

Servings: 2

Ingredients:

- 1 8-oz boneless, skin on trout fillet
- 2 cups chicken broth or water
- 2 leeks, halved
- 6-8 slices lemon
- salt and pepper to taste

Directions:

1. On medium fire, place a large nonstick skillet and arrange leeks and lemons on pan in a layer. Cover with soup stock or water and bring to a simmer.
2. Meanwhile, season trout on both sides with pepper and salt. Place trout on simmering pan of water. Cover and cook until trout is flaky, around 8 minutes.
3. In a serving platter, spoon leek and lemons on bottom of plate, top with trout and spoon sauce into plate. Serve and enjoy.

Nutrition: Calories: 360.2; Protein: 13.8g; Fat: 7.5g; Carbs: 51.5g

41. Leftover Salmon Salad Power Bowls

Preparation Time: 10 minutes

Cooking Time: 10 minutes

Servings: 1

Ingredients:

- ½ cup raspberries
- ½ cup zucchini, sliced
- 1 lemon, juice squeezed
- 1 tbsp. balsamic glaze
- 2 sprigs of thyme, chopped
- 2 tbsp. olive oil
- 4 cups seasonal greens
- 4 oz. leftover grilled salmon
- Salt and pepper to taste

Directions:

1. Heat oil in a skillet over medium flame and sauté the zucchini. Season with salt and pepper to taste.
2. In a mixing bowl, mix all ingredients together.
3. Toss to combine everything.
4. Sprinkle with nut cheese.

Nutrition: Calories: 450.3; Fat: 35.5 g; Protein: 23.4g; Carbs: 9.3 g

APPETIZER AND SNACK RECIPES

42. Date Wraps

Preparation time: 10 minutes

Cooking time: 0 minutes

Servings: 8

Ingredients:

- 8 whole dates, pitted
- 8 thin slices prosciutto
- Freshly ground pepper to taste

Directions:

1. Take one date and one slice prosciutto. Wrap the prosciutto around the dates and place on a serving platter. Garnish with pepper and serve.

Nutrition: Calories 35 Fat 1 g Carbohydrate 6 g Protein 2 g

43. Clementine & Pistachio Ricotta

Preparation time: 5 minutes

Cooking time: 0 minutes

Servings: 2

Ingredients:

- 2/3 cup part-skim ricotta
- 2 clementine's, peeled, separated into segments, deseeded
- 4 teaspoons chopped pistachio nuts

Directions:

1. Place 1/3 cup ricotta in each of 2 bowls. Divide the clementine segments equally and place over the ricotta. Sprinkle pistachio nuts on top and serve.

Nutrition: Calories 178 Fat 9 g Carbohydrate 15 g Protein 11 g

44. Serrano-Wrapped Plums

Preparation time: 10 minutes

Cooking time: 0 minutes

Servings: 4

Ingredients:

- 2 firm ripe plums or peaches or nectarines, quartered
- 1 ounce thinly sliced Serrano ham or prosciutto or jamón Ibérico, cut into 8 pieces

Directions:

1. Take one piece of ham and one piece of fruit. Wrap the ham around the fruit and place on a serving platter. Serve.

Nutrition: Calories 30 Fat 1 g Carbohydrate 4 g Protein 2 g

DESSERT RECIPES

45. Italian Bean Soup

Preparation Time: 15 minutes

Cooking Time: 15 minutes

Servings: 2

Ingredients:

- 1 tablespoon virgin olive oil
- 1 onion (diced)
- 2 garlic cloves (minced)
- 2 cups tomato sauce (homemade or 1 can of low-sodium organic canned tomato sauce)
- 3 cups cooked cannellini beans (or about 24 ounces of canned beans that have been drained and rinsed)
- 1 tablespoon basil (dried)
- ½ teaspoon oregano
- ¼ teaspoon black pepper

Directions:

1. Take a large soup or stockpot and place it on your stove. Turn the heat all the way up to medium-high and pour in the virgin olive oil.
2. Allow the oil to heat slightly before adding your diced onions to the pot. Sautee for 3 minutes and then adds the garlic. Let the flavors come together for 2 minutes.

3. Add the cannellini beans, basil, oregano, and black pepper to the pot. Stir everything together then pour over the tomato sauce.
4. Allow the sauce to come to a steady simmer. Reduce the heat to medium-low. Cover your pot so the flavors can simmer together for 5 minutes.
5. Uncover the pot and allow the aroma to fill your kitchen. Then, take a ladle and fill your soup bowls! Grab a soup spoon and enjoy

Nutrition: Calories – 164, Carbs - 25.6 g, Protein - 8.1 g, Fat - 3.8 g

46. Red Soup, Seville Style

Preparation Time: 15 minutes

Cooking Time: 15 minutes

Servings: 2

Ingredients:

- 2 ounces stale bread, crusts removed
- 3 tablespoons further virgin olive oil
- 3 tablespoons fortified wine vinegar
- 2 garlic cloves, crushed
- 2 teaspoon salt
- teaspoon cayenne pepper pinch of cumin
- little red onion, chopped
- pound ripe tomatoes, peeled, seeded, and chopped
- cucumber, peeled, seeded, and chopped
- red peppers, cored, seeded, and chopped
- cups ice water
- For the garnish:
- 4 tablespoons red peppers, cored, seeded, and finely chopped
- 4 tablespoons finely cut cucumber
- 4 tablespoons finely cut purple onion
- 2 tablespoons finely cut contemporary mint leaves

Directions

1. First of all, you should Soak the bread into water and after that squeeze dry.
2. Place in a blender or kitchen appliance

3. with the vegetable oil, vinegar, garlic, salt, and spices and method to a sleek cream.
4. Add the onion, tomatoes, cucumber, and peppers and 1/2 the drinking water and still method the vegetables till sleek.
5. Pour into a soup serving dish and add the remaining water.
6. Chill totally before serving. Place the garnishes in little dishes and serve with the soup.

Nutrition: Calories: 123, Fats: 3g, Dietary Fiber: 5g, Carbohydrates: 19g, Protein: 5g

47. Garlic Soup

Preparation Time: 15 minutes

Cooking Time: 0 minutes

Servings: 2

Ingredients:

- 5 cups water
- head garlic, unpeeled
- sprigs fresh thyme
- tablespoons further virgin olive oil
- Salt
- Freshly ground black pepper
- 2 egg yolks
- slices of bread, gently toasted

Directions

1. Bring the water to boil with the garlic and thyme and simmer for twenty minutes.
2. Take away the garlic and peel. Place the flesh in an exceedingly bowl and mash with a fork.
3. Step by step add the vegetable oil and blend well. Return to the soup.
4. Take away the thyme and after that you should Season it with salt & black pepper.
5. Beat the egg yolks in another bowl and step by step add a ladleful of the soup.

6. Combine well and stir into the soup. Simmer for some minutes, however don't let it boil or the soup can curdle.
7. Place the slices of toasts in individual bowls and pour over the soup. Serve at once.

Nutrition: Calories: 123, Fats: 3g, Dietary Fiber: 5g, Carbohydrates: 19g, Protein: 5g

48. Dalmatian Cabbage, Potato, And Pea Soup

Preparation Time: 15 minutes

Cooking Time: 15 minutes

Servings: 2

Ingredients:

- 4 tablespoons further virgin olive oil
- medium onion, chopped
- carrots, coarsely grated
- medium potatoes, peeled and diced into little items inexperienced cabbage, shredded
- cup contemporary shelled peas, or frozen petit pois
- quart water
- Salt
- Freshly ground black pepper

Directions

1. Heat the vegetable oil in an exceedingly massive pot and cook the onion over a moderate heat for three minutes.
2. Add the carrots, potatoes, and cabbage and still cook for an additional five minutes.
3. Add the peas and water and produce to a boil.
4. Cowl and simmer for thirty-five to forty minutes or till the vegetables are tender and also the soup is fairly thick.

5. Finally, you must season it with salt & black pepper and serve hot.

Nutrition: Calories: 123, Fats: 3g, Dietary Fiber: 5g, Carbohydrates: 19g, Protein: 5g

49. Mini Nuts and Fruits Crumble

Preparation time: 15 minutes

Cooking time: 15 minutes

Servings: 6

Ingredients:

- Topping:
- ¼ cup coarsely chopped hazelnuts
- 1 cup coarsely chopped walnuts
- 1 teaspoon ground cinnamon
- Sea salt, to taste
- 1 tablespoon melted coconut oil
- Filling:
- 6 fresh figs, quartered
- 2 nectarines, pitted and sliced
- 1 cup fresh blueberries
- 2 teaspoons lemon zest
- ½ cup raw honey
- 1 teaspoon vanilla extract

Directions:

1. Combine the ingredients for the topping in a bowl. Stir to mix well. Set aside until ready to use.
2. Preheat the oven to 375ºF (190ºC). Combine the ingredients for the fillings in a bowl. Stir to mix well. Divide the filling in six ramekins, then divide and top with nut topping.

3. Bake in the preheated oven for 15 minutes or until the topping is lightly browned and the filling is frothy. Serve immediately.

Nutrition: Calories: 336 Fat: 18.8g Protein: 6.3g Carbs: 41.9g

50. Mint Banana Chocolate Sorbet

Preparation time: 4 hours & 5 minutes

Cooking time: 0 minutes

Servings: 1

Ingredients:

- 1 frozen banana
- 1 tablespoon almond butter
- 2 tablespoons minced fresh mint
- 2 to 3 tablespoons dark chocolate chips (60% cocoa or higher)
- 2 to 3 tablespoons goji (optional)

Directions:

1. Put the banana, butter, and mint in a food processor. Pulse to purée until creamy and smooth. Add the chocolate and goji, then pulse for several more times to combine well.
2. Pour the mixture in a bowl or a ramekin, then freeze for at least 4 hours before serving chilled.

Nutrition: Calories: 213 Fat: 9.8g Protein: 3.1g Carbs: 2.9g

Lightning Source UK Ltd.
Milton Keynes UK
UKHW020813150321
380363UK00001B/10